Rosie and the Worry Whisperer

Matthew Cunningham (text)

Katharine Hall (illustrations)

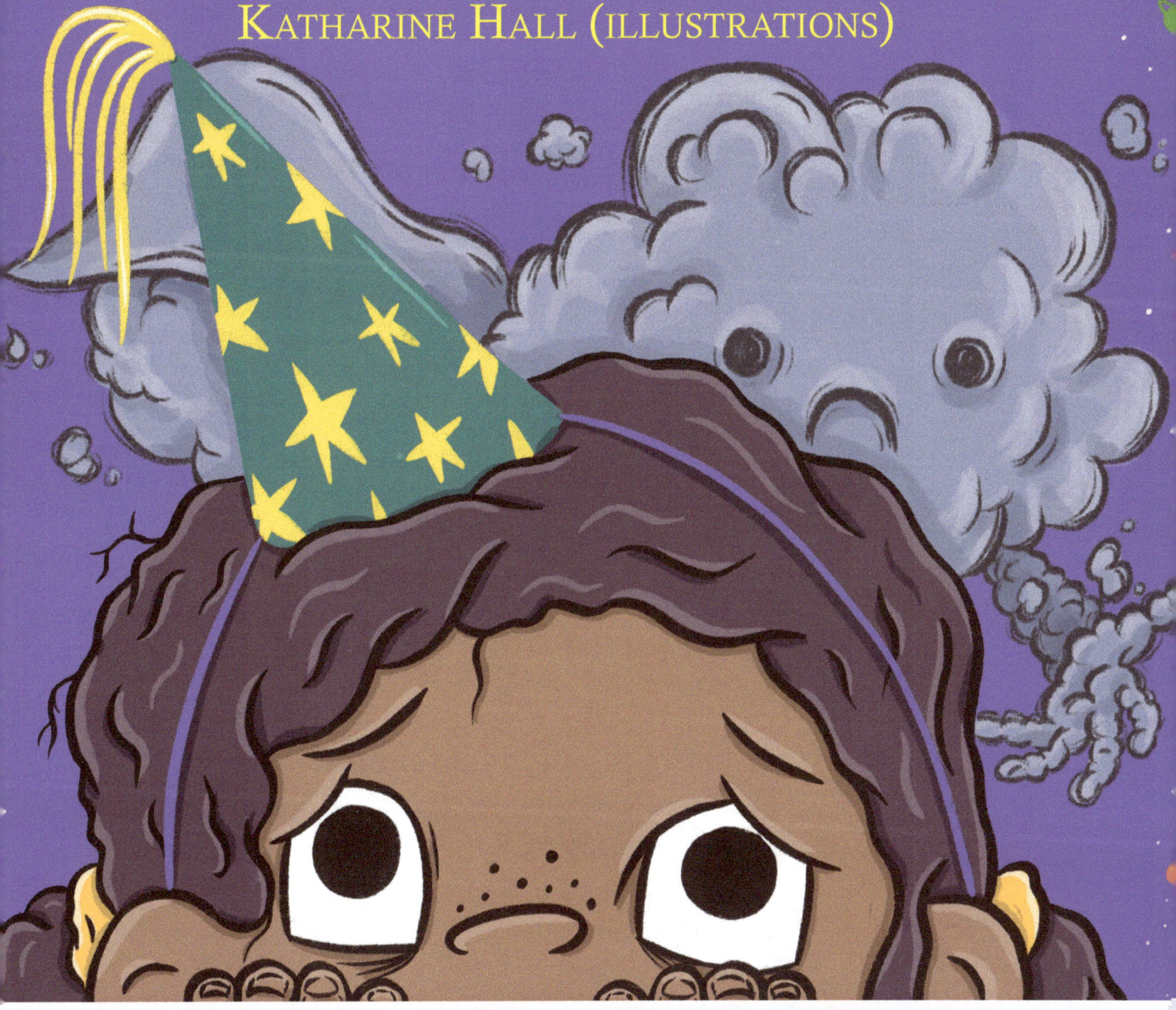

Rosie wakes with the sun.

It is a big day. She is six years old –
almost a grown-up, she thinks.

FRom
AMELIA

Her birthday party is at the space museum tonight.
They have a planetarium, some moon rocks, and a
telescope as big as her bedroom. She can think of
nowhere more exciting to have her party.

But her worry whisperer isn't so sure.

WHAT IF THERE ARE TOO MANY PEOPLE THERE? it whispers.

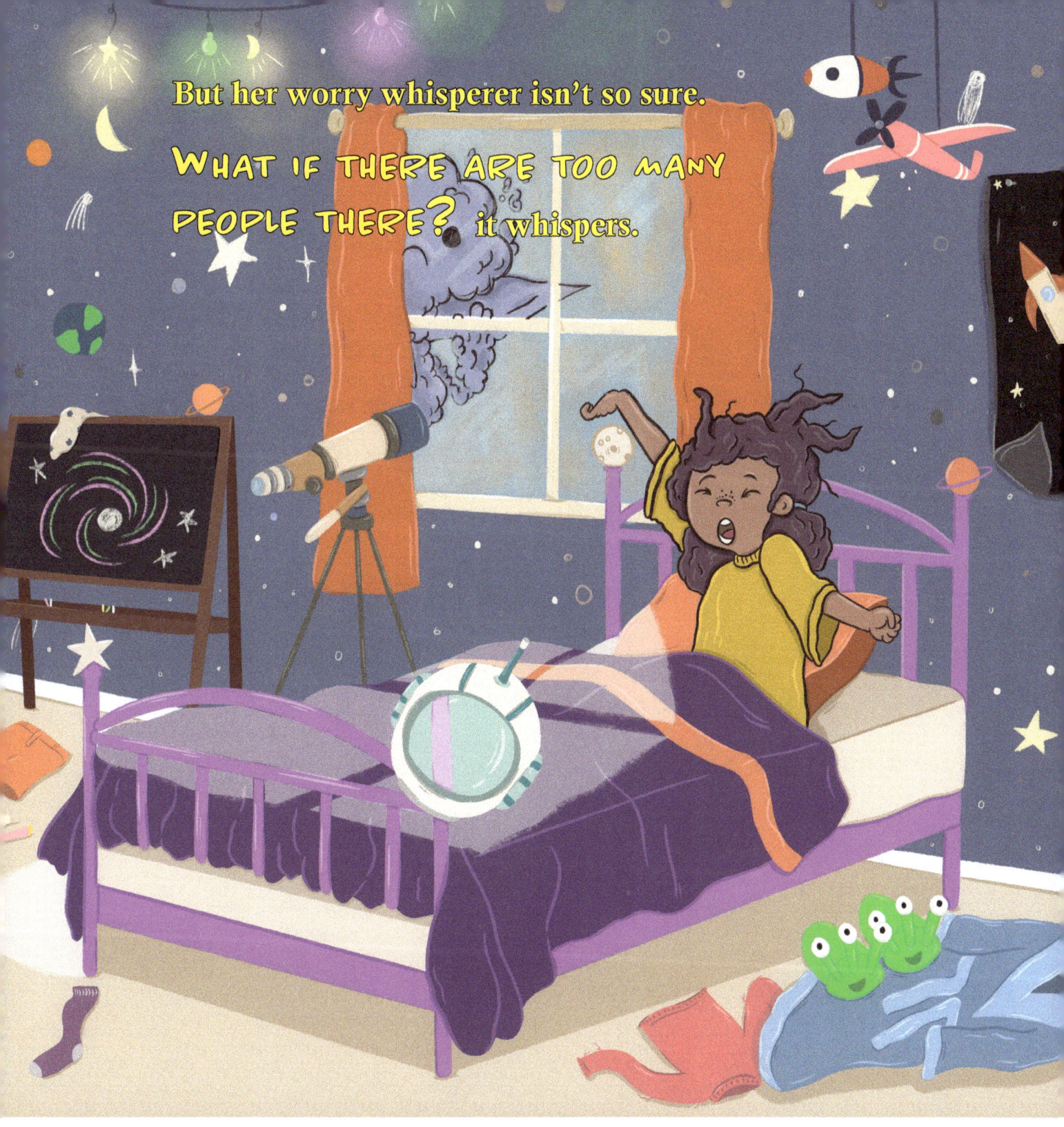

Rosie thinks about this while she eats her breakfast.
She thinks a lot about what her worry whisperer tells her –
even when she doesn't want to.

"Daddy," she asks, "will there be lots of people
at my party?"

"Just your friends from school," he answers.

"But what about other kids?" Rosie asks.
"Will there be other parties tonight?"

"Maybe," Daddy says, slurping his coffee.

"Oh." Her worry whisperer doesn't like the sound of that.

Being around lots of people makes her feel really small,
even though Daddy says she is growing every day.

"It will be fun," says Daddy, patting her arm gently.
"I promise."

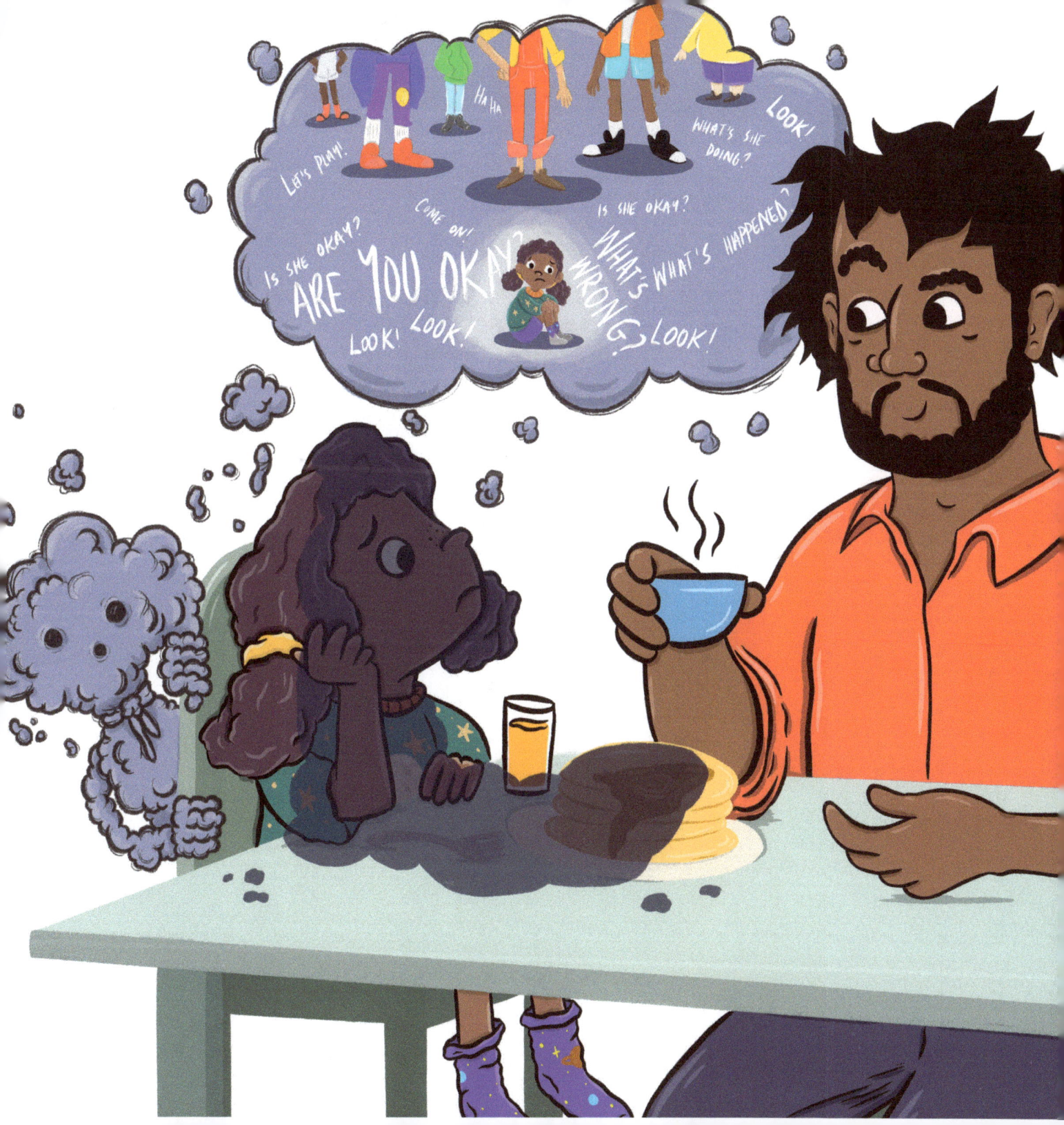

WHAT IF IT RAINS, AND NOBODY COMES?

says Rosie's worry whisperer on the way to the party.

She thinks of what it would feel like to have a birthday party with no friends. It makes her sad.

Her worry whisperer often makes her feel sad.

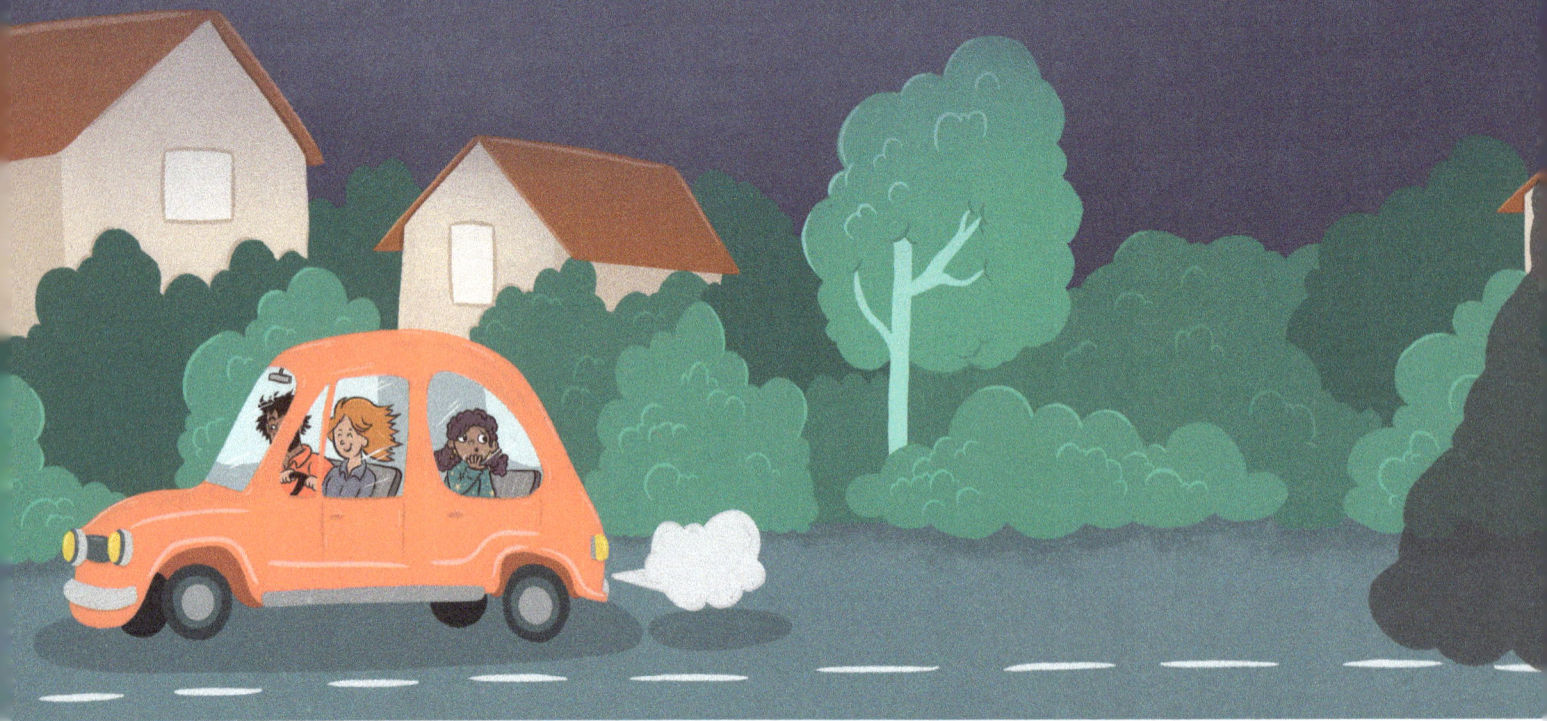

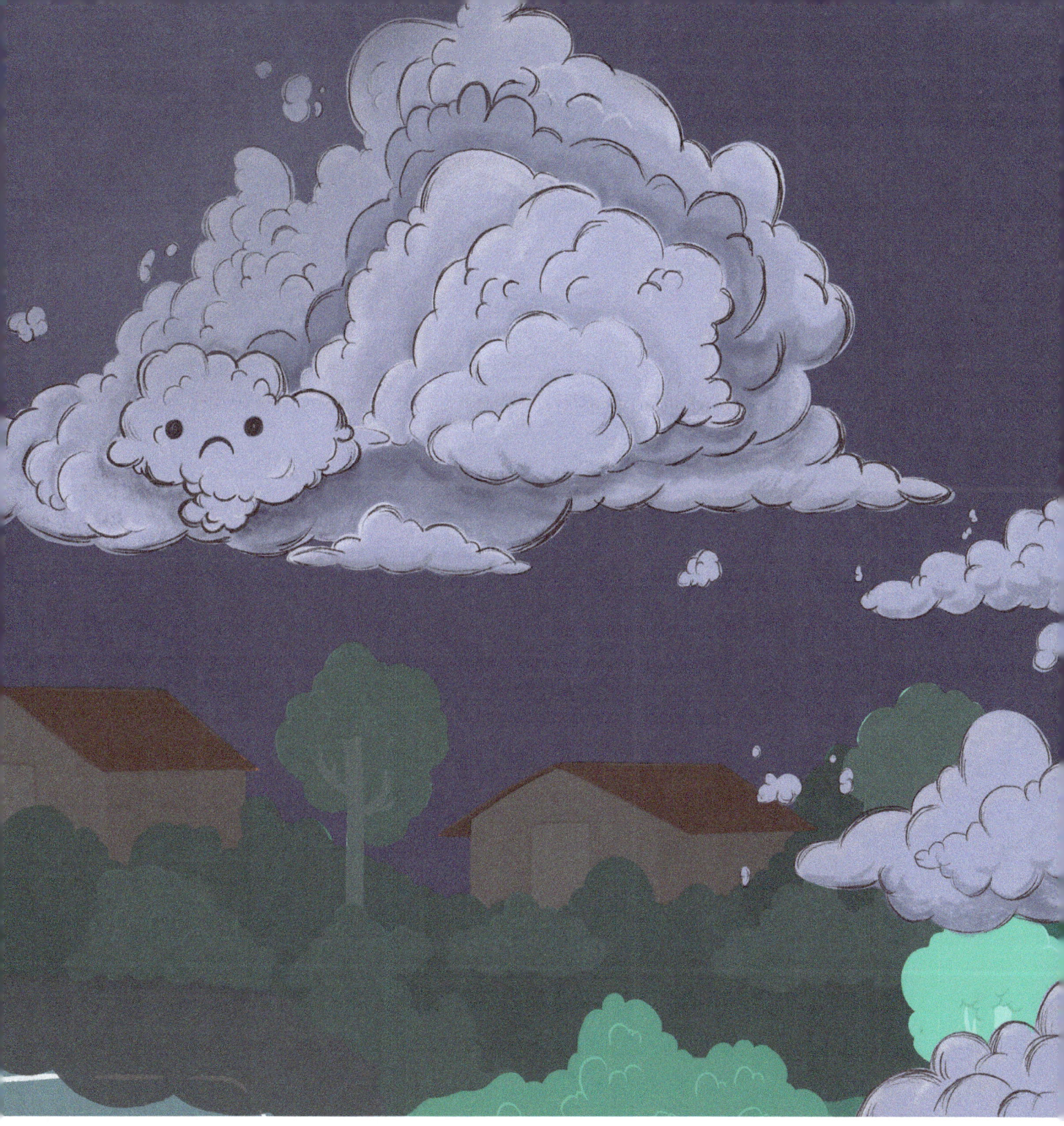

Mummy and Daddy help set up the tables and the food at the space museum.

Rosie keeps checking the entrance to see if her friends have arrived.

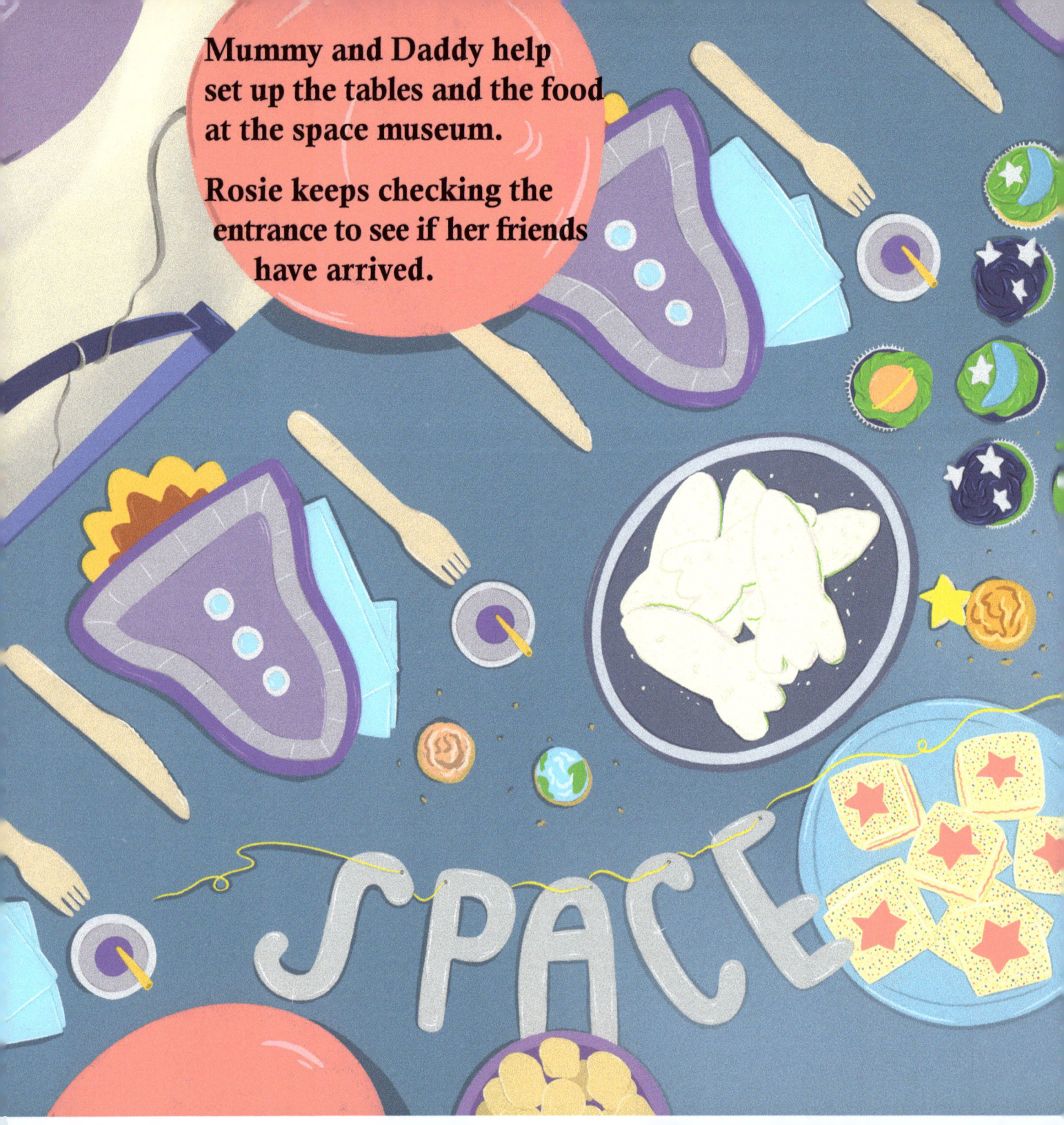

"Amelia is here!" says Rosie.

Amelia gives Rosie a big present wrapped in astronaut wrapping paper, and a home-made card.

"It says 'to my best friend', because you're my best friend, Rosie!"

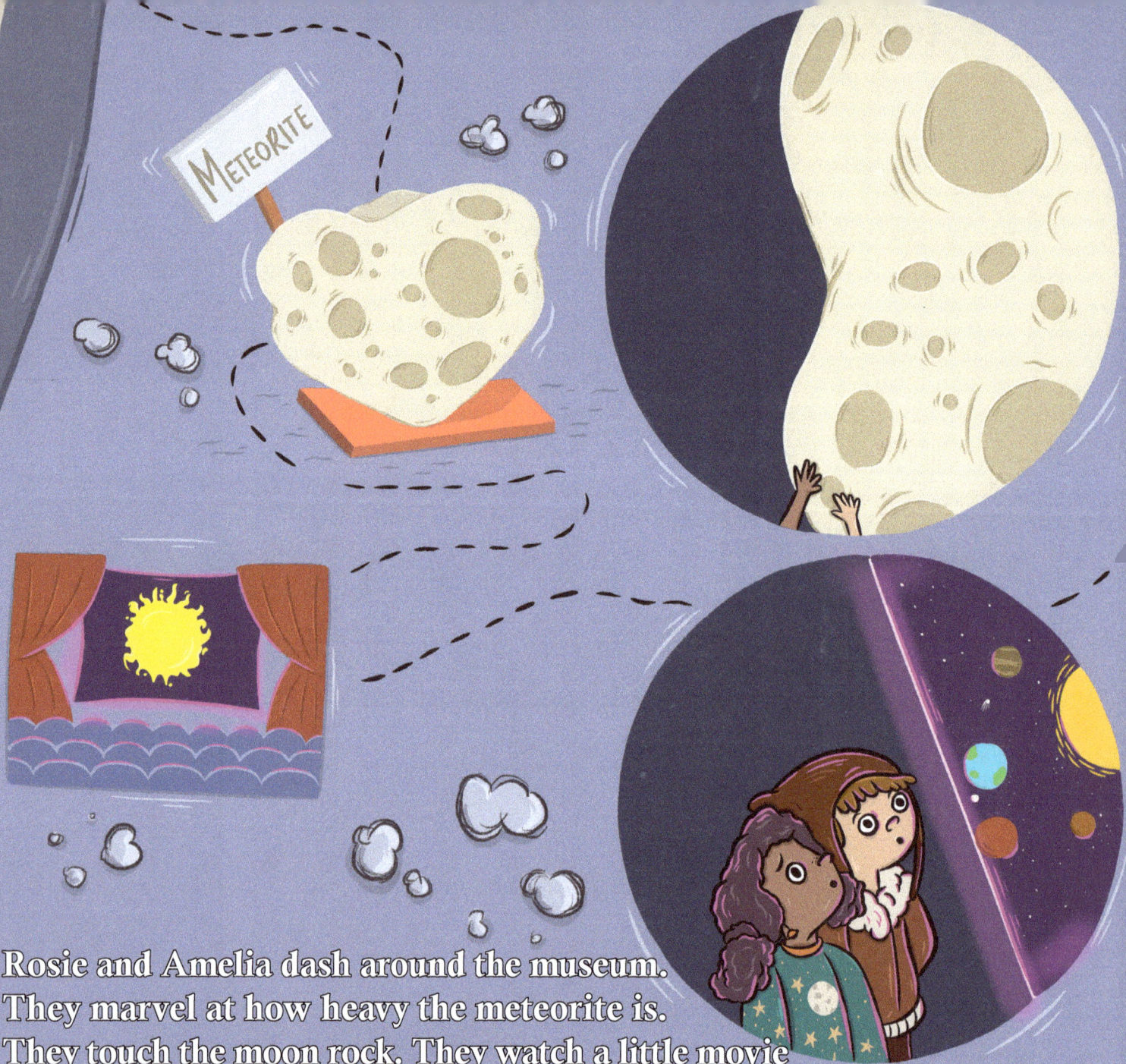

Rosie and Amelia dash around the museum.
They marvel at how heavy the meteorite is.
They touch the moon rock. They watch a little movie
about where the Sun and the planets came from.

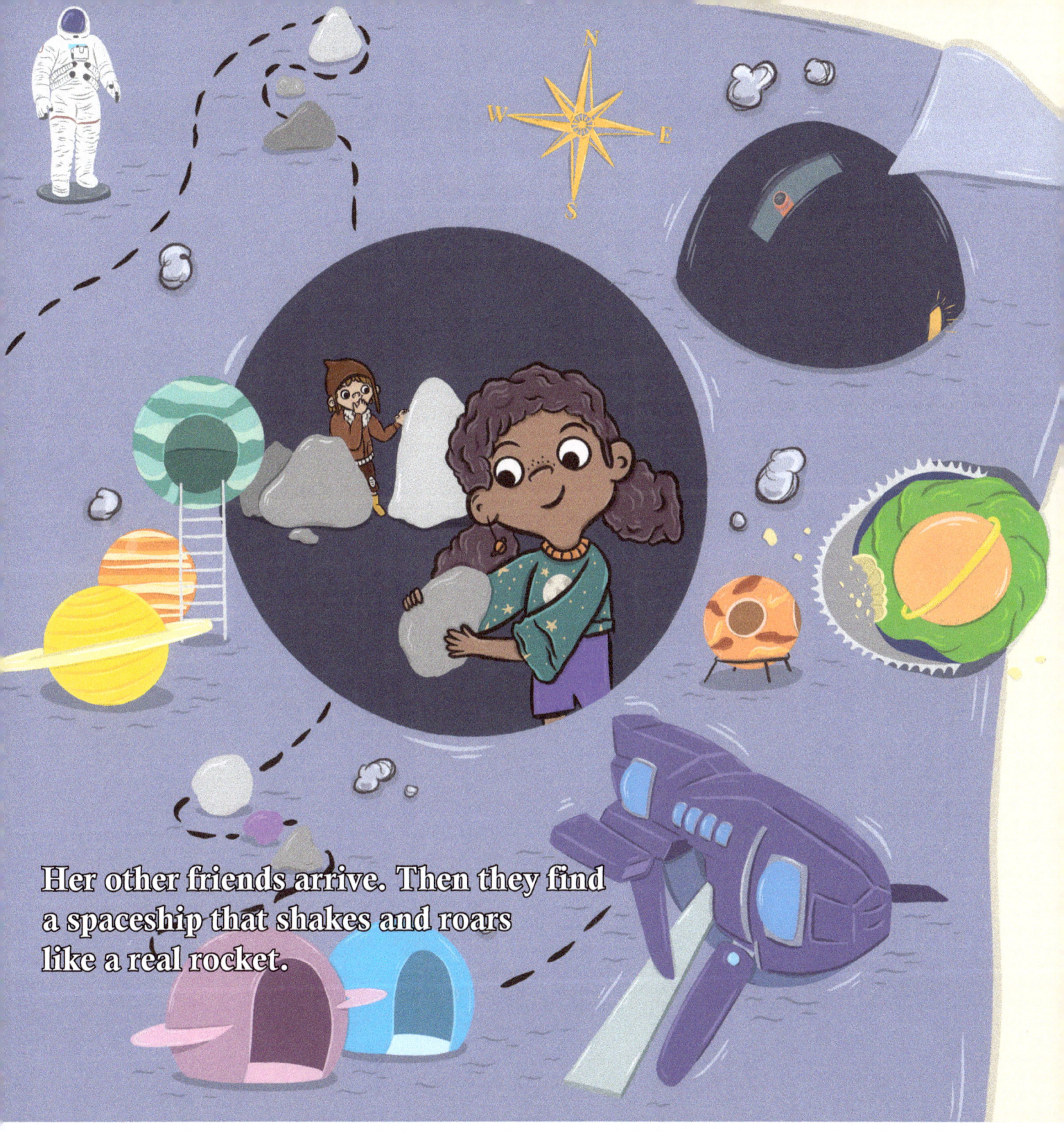

Her other friends arrive. Then they find a spaceship that shakes and roars like a real rocket.

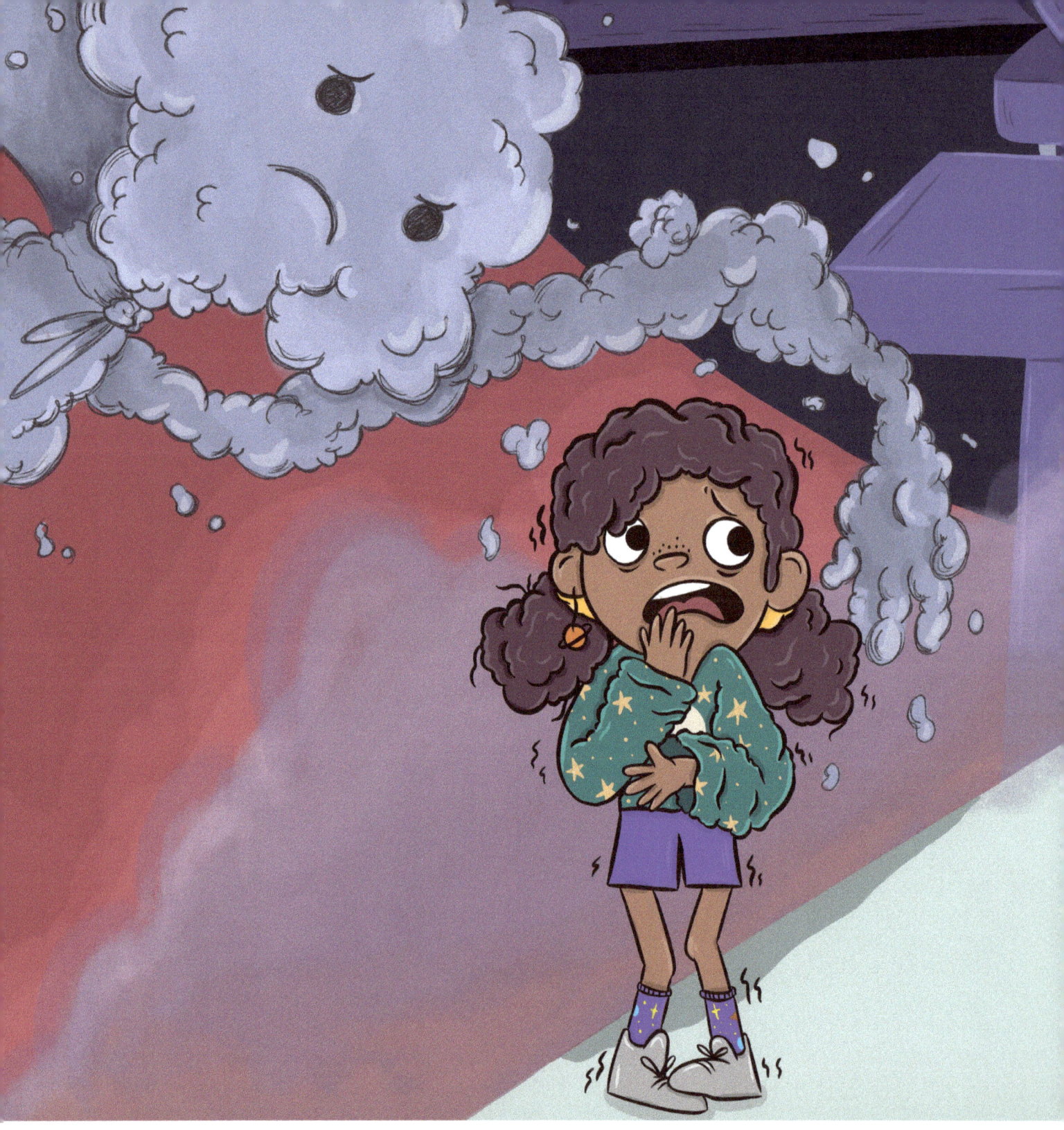

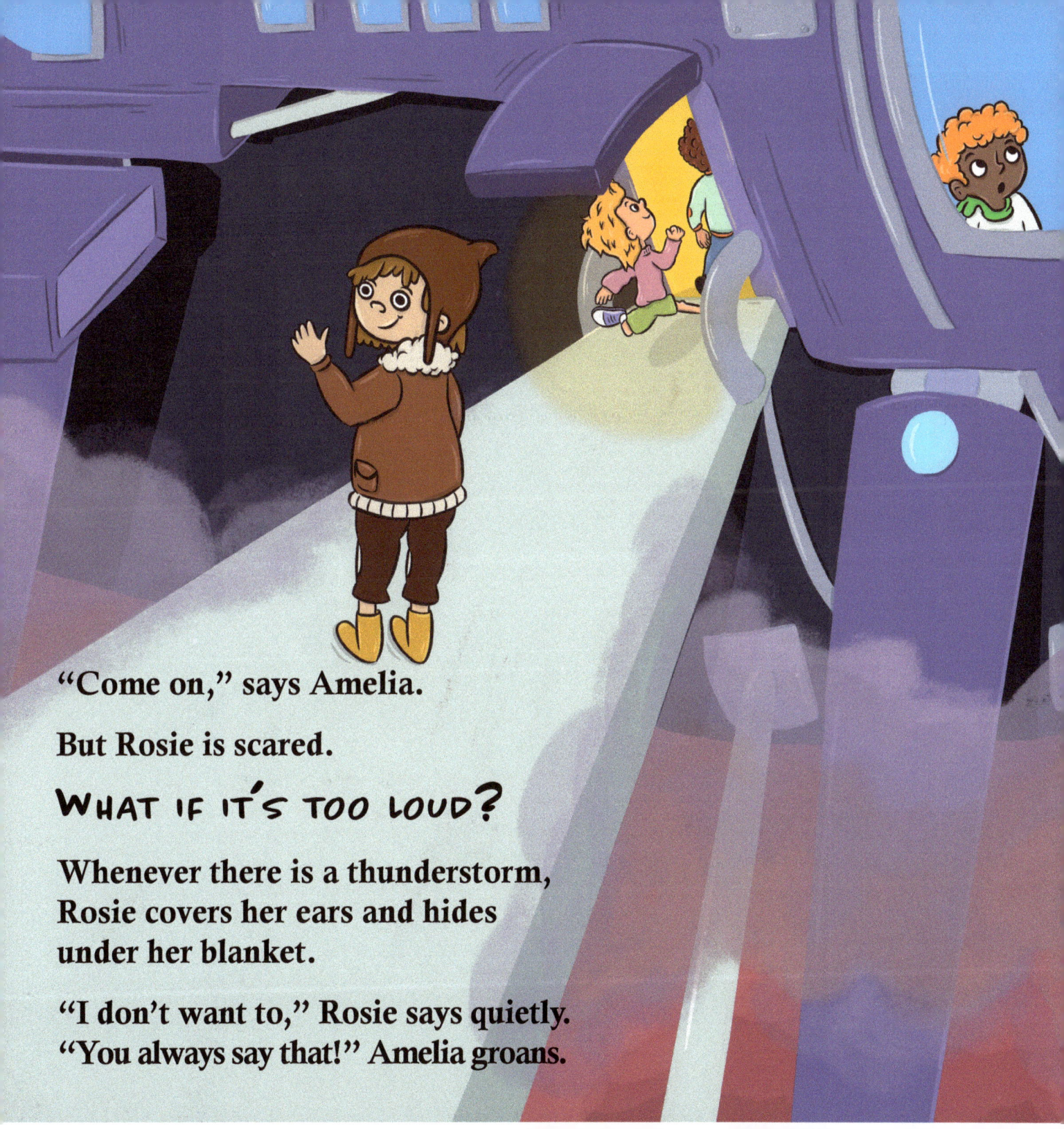

"Come on," says Amelia.

But Rosie is scared.

WHAT IF IT'S TOO LOUD?

Whenever there is a thunderstorm, Rosie covers her ears and hides under her blanket.

"I don't want to," Rosie says quietly. "You always say that!" Amelia groans.

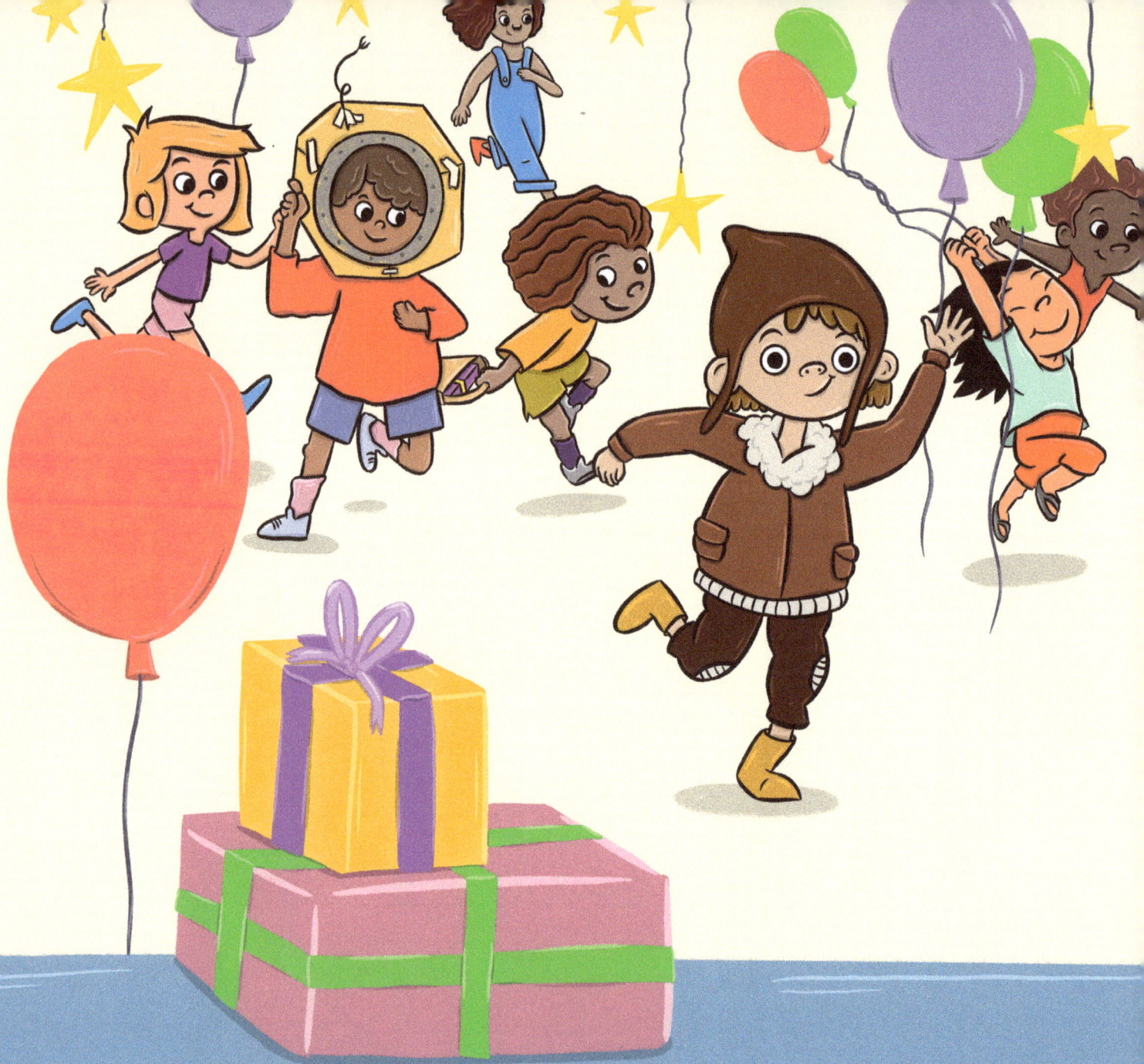

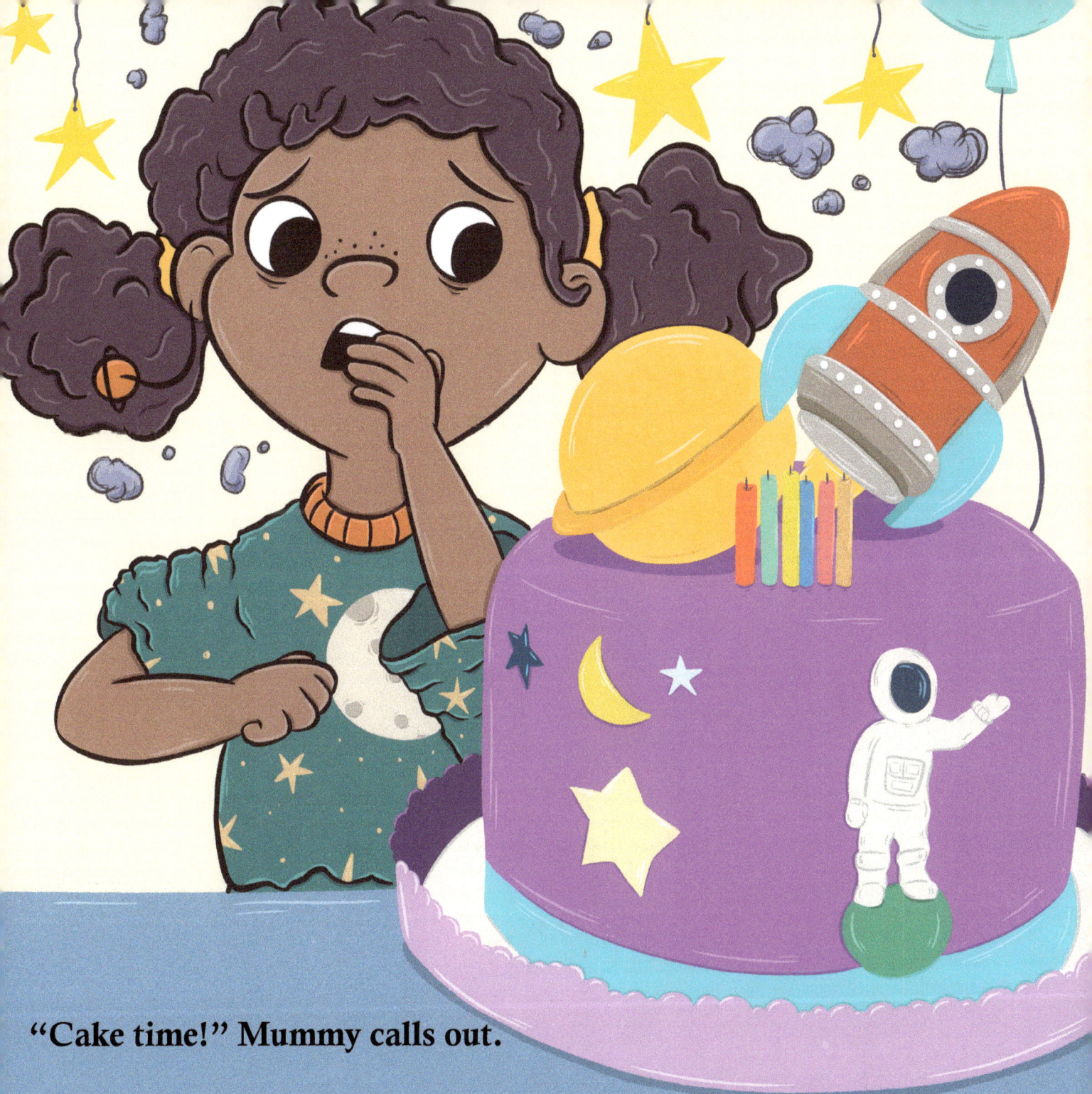

"Cake time!" Mummy calls out.

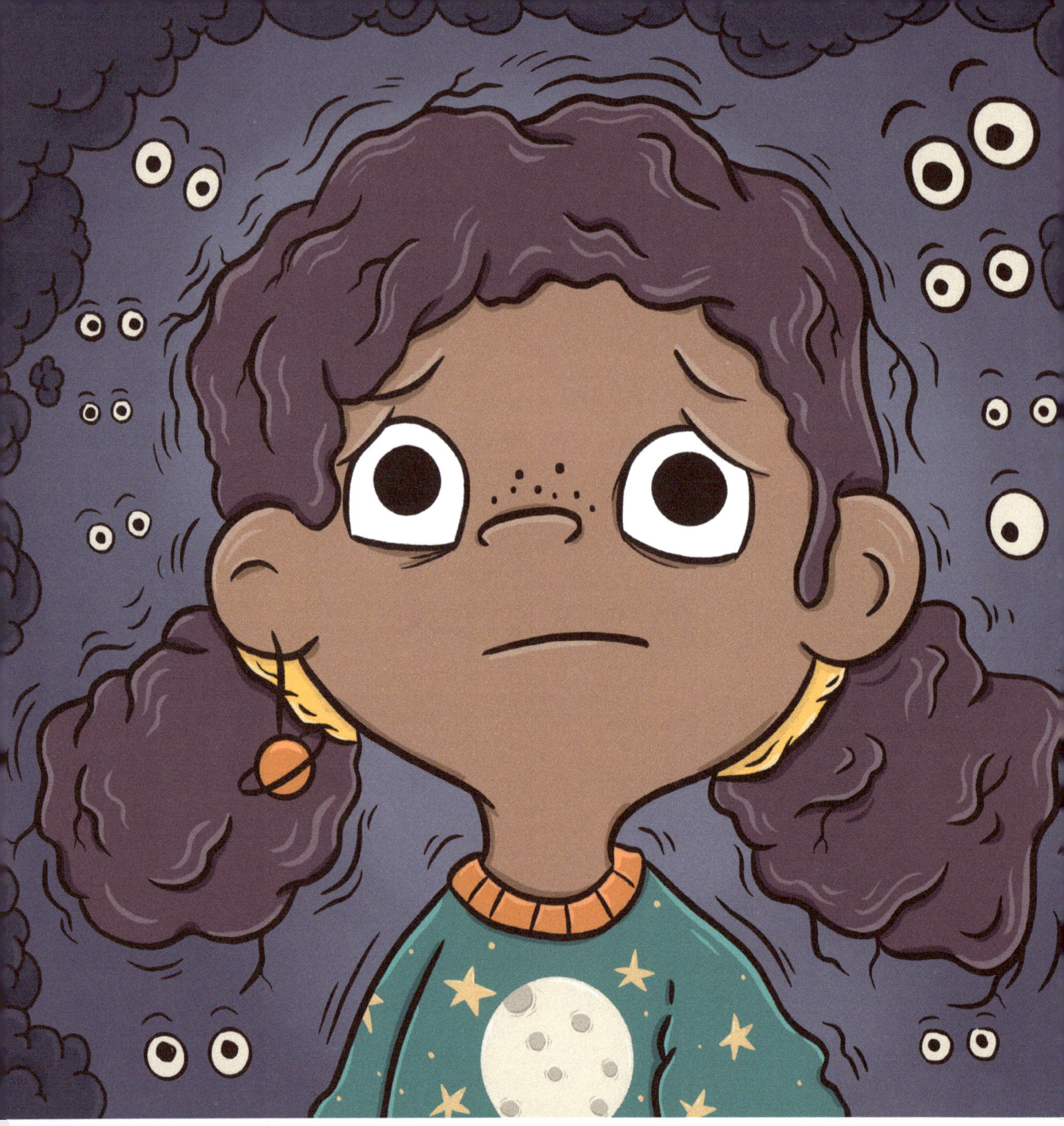

Rosie sits in a special rocket chair at the head of the table. Everyone is watching her – friends, mummies and daddies. More people than Rosie can count, and she can count really high. Her tummy is gurgling, and her heart is thumping.

I DON'T LIKE THIS,
her worry whisperer says.

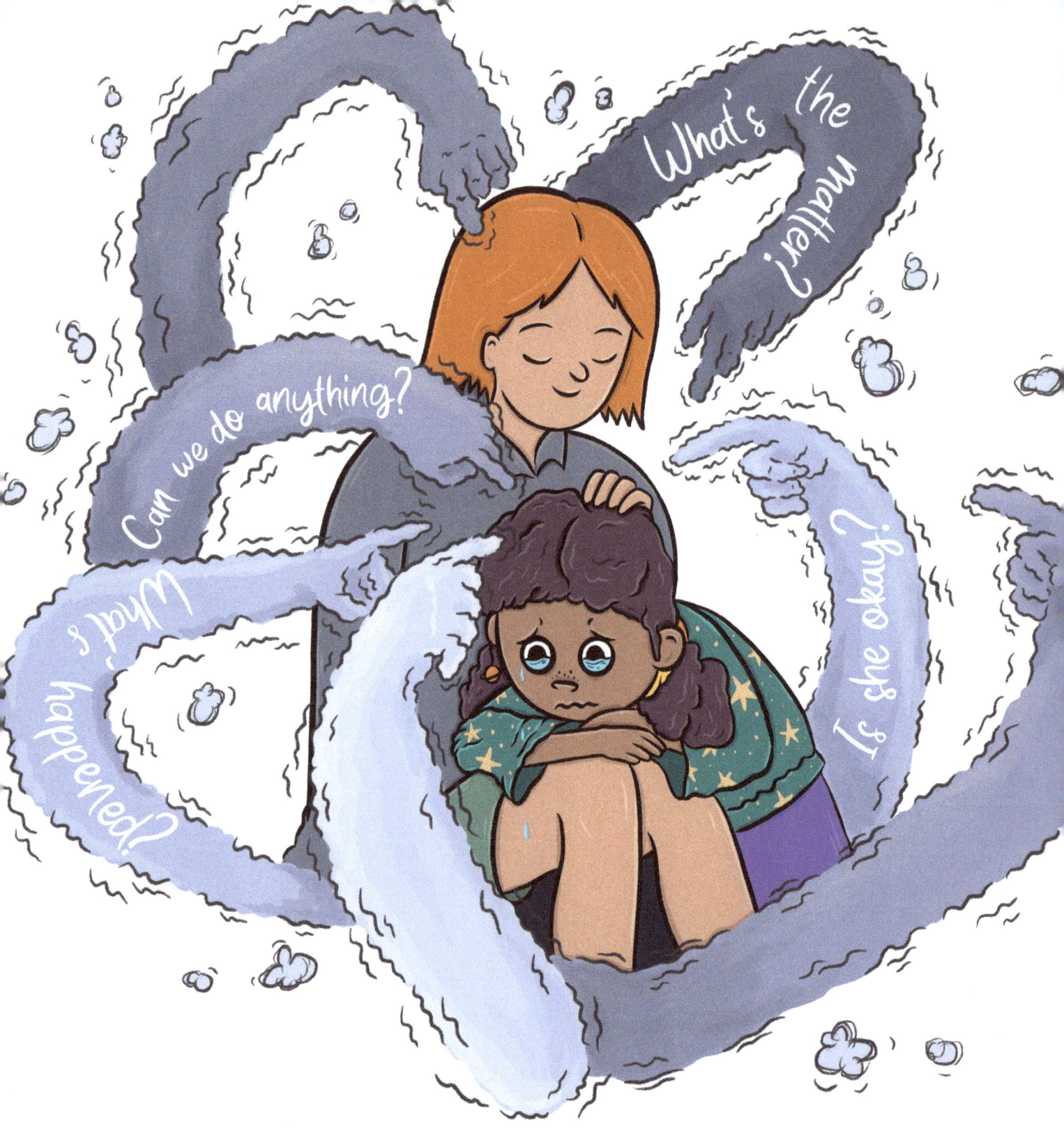

Before they can finish singing 'Happy Birthday',
Rosie begins to cry.

Voices buzz around her head
like bumblebees.

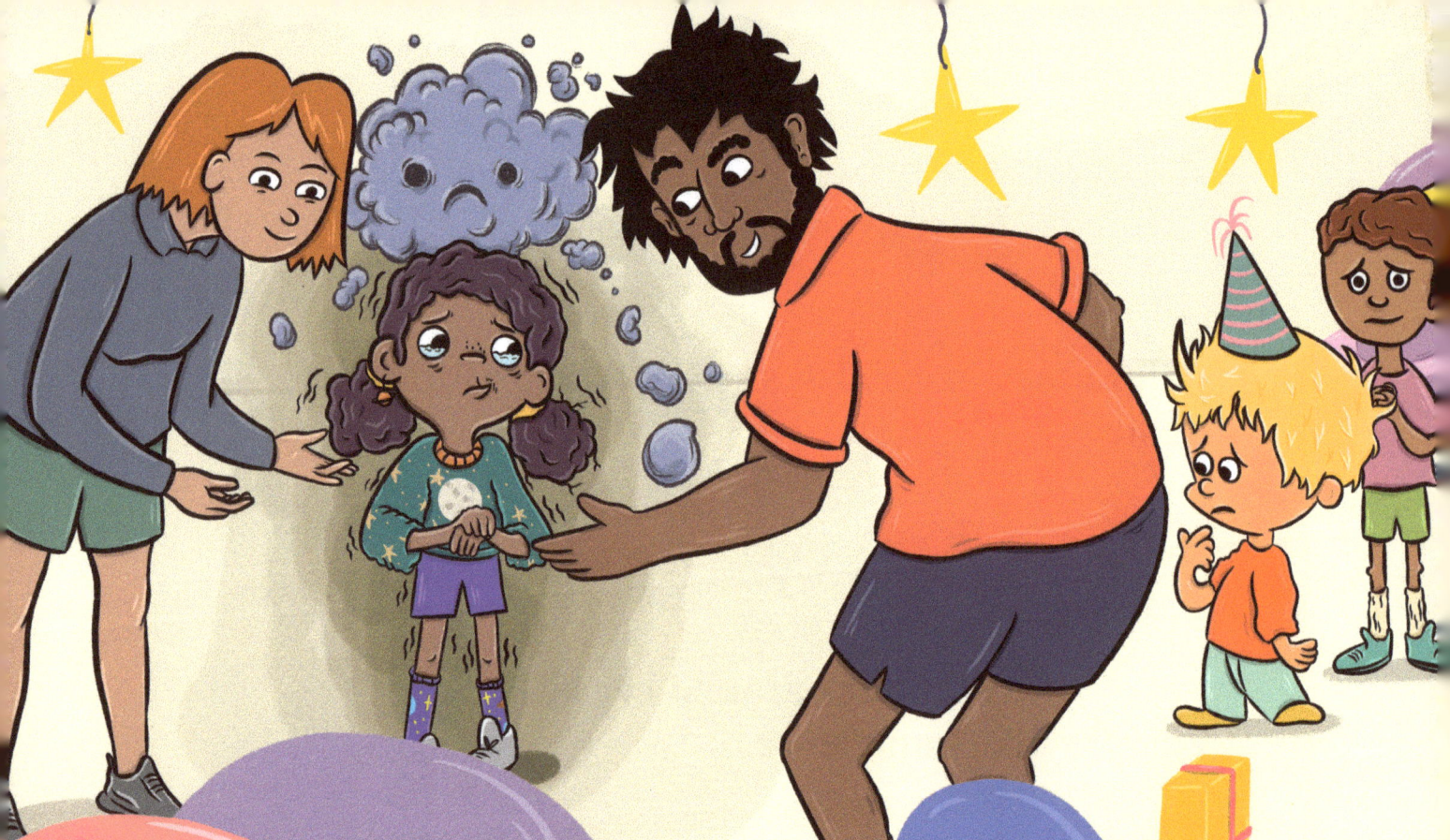

"Sweetheart," Mummy asks, "do you want to tell us what upset you?"

"I don't know," Rosie whimpers. Sometimes she finds it hard to describe how she feels.

"It's okay to cry sometimes," Mummy says. "Even mummies and daddies cry. But it's also important to try to be brave."

Daddy takes her hand. "Come with us. We have a surprise for you, Rosie."

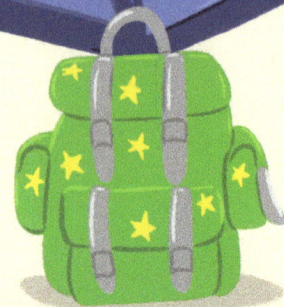

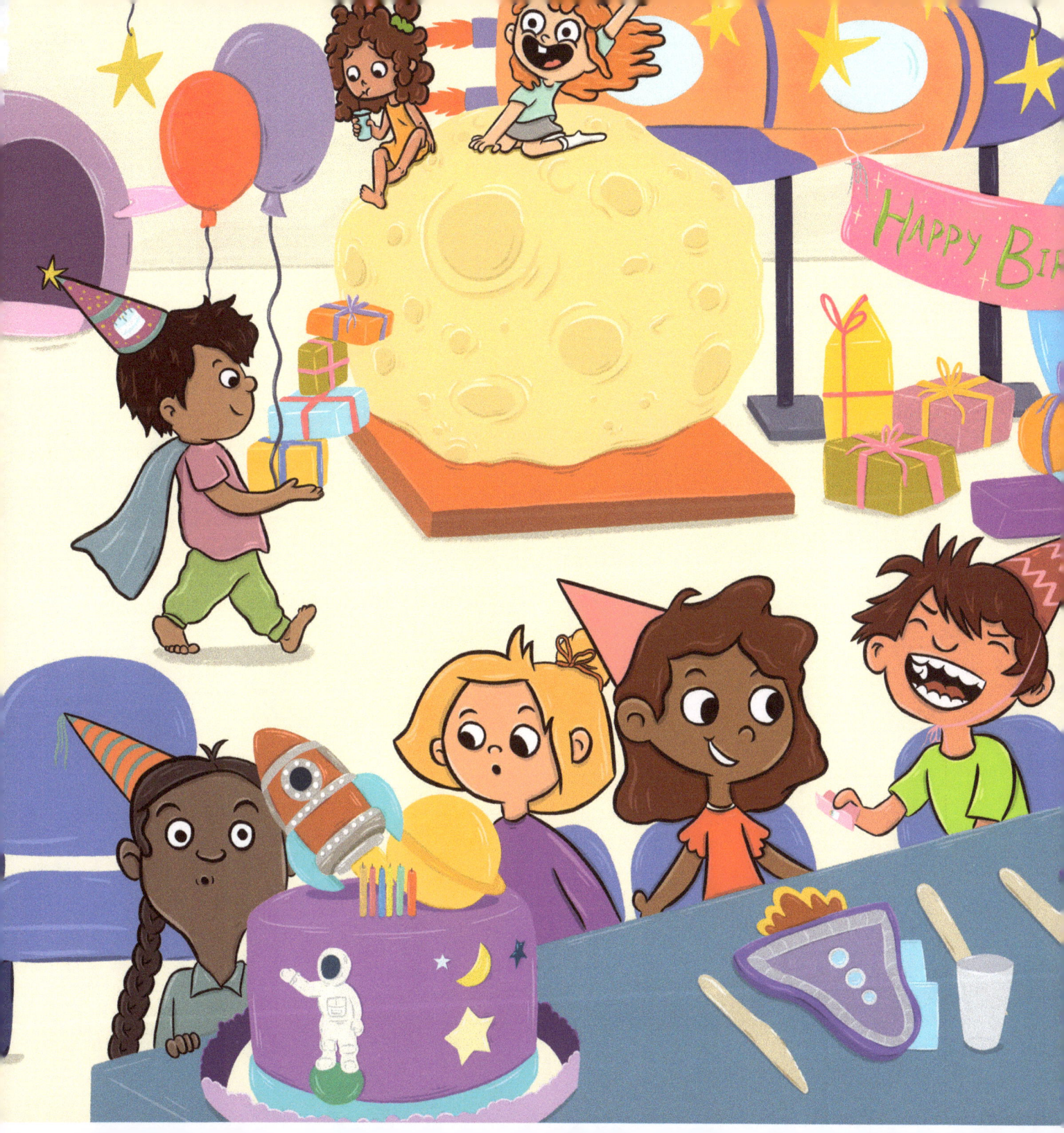

HAPPY BI

In the star dome is the biggest telescope Rosie has ever seen.

"Go on," Daddy says, "take a look."

The night sky feels like it is pushing down on her.

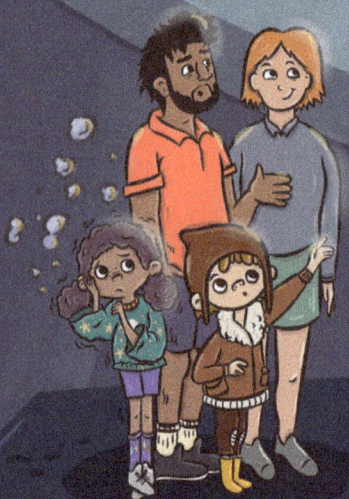

WHAT IF IT'S SCARY?
WHAT IF THE DARKNESS
SWALLOWS YOU UP?

Her worry whisperer is loud
and demanding.

"I don't want to!" she cries.

"I get scared too, you know," Daddy admits gently.
"Sometimes it feels like there is a voice in my head,
telling me not to do things, or not to try things.
Do you hear that too?"

Rosie nods.

"That voice is your protector," Daddy says.
"It wants to keeps you safe. But sometimes,
it does its job too well. Sometimes we need
to remind it that we don't always
need protection."

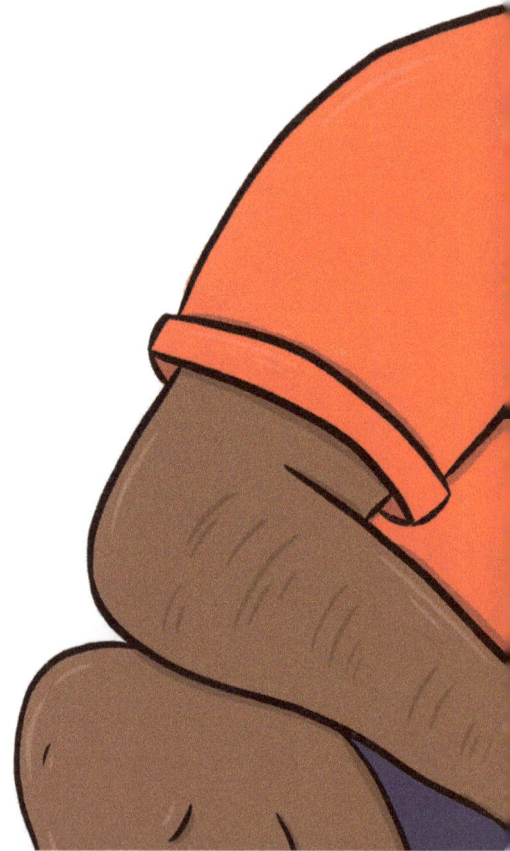

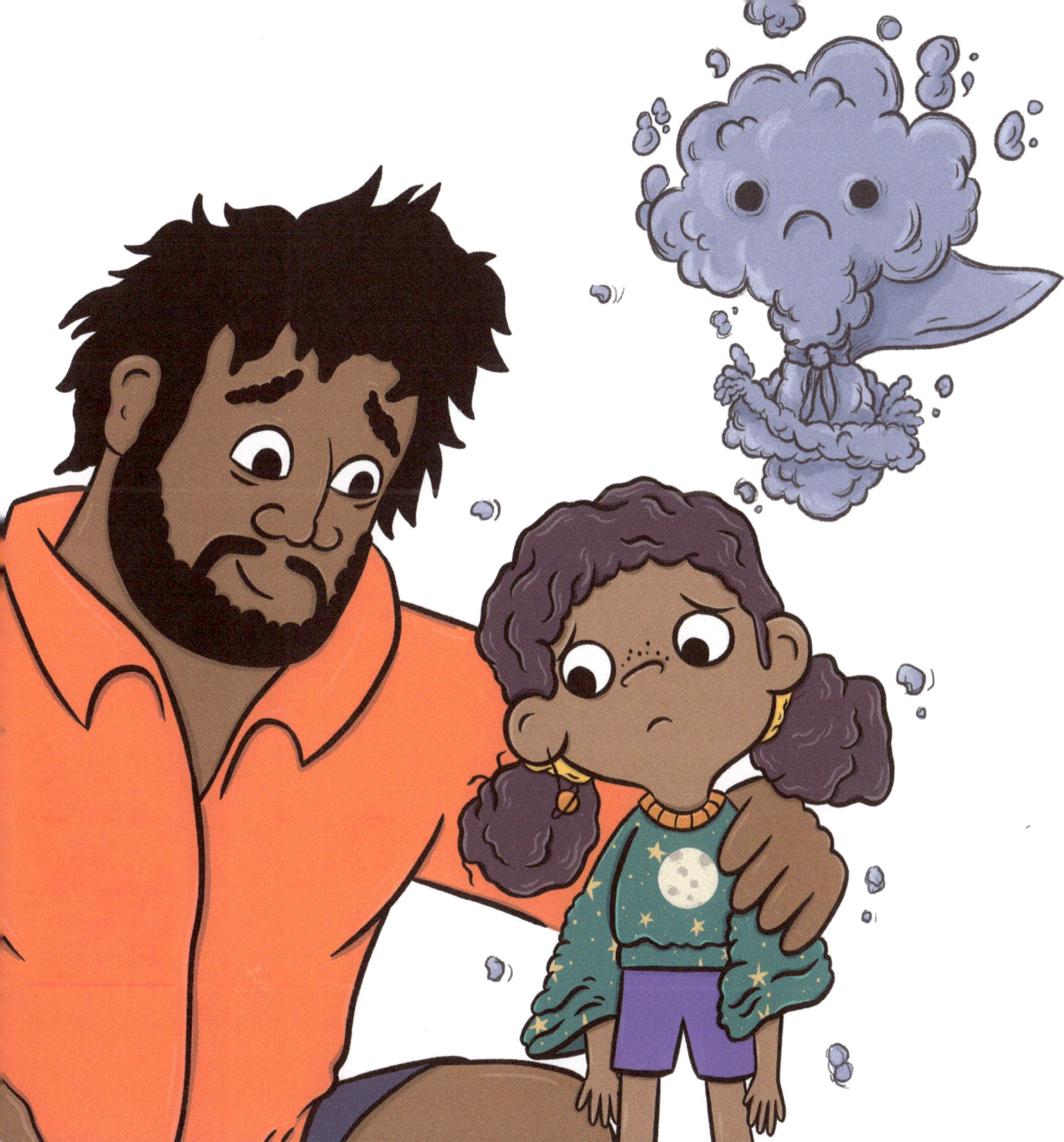

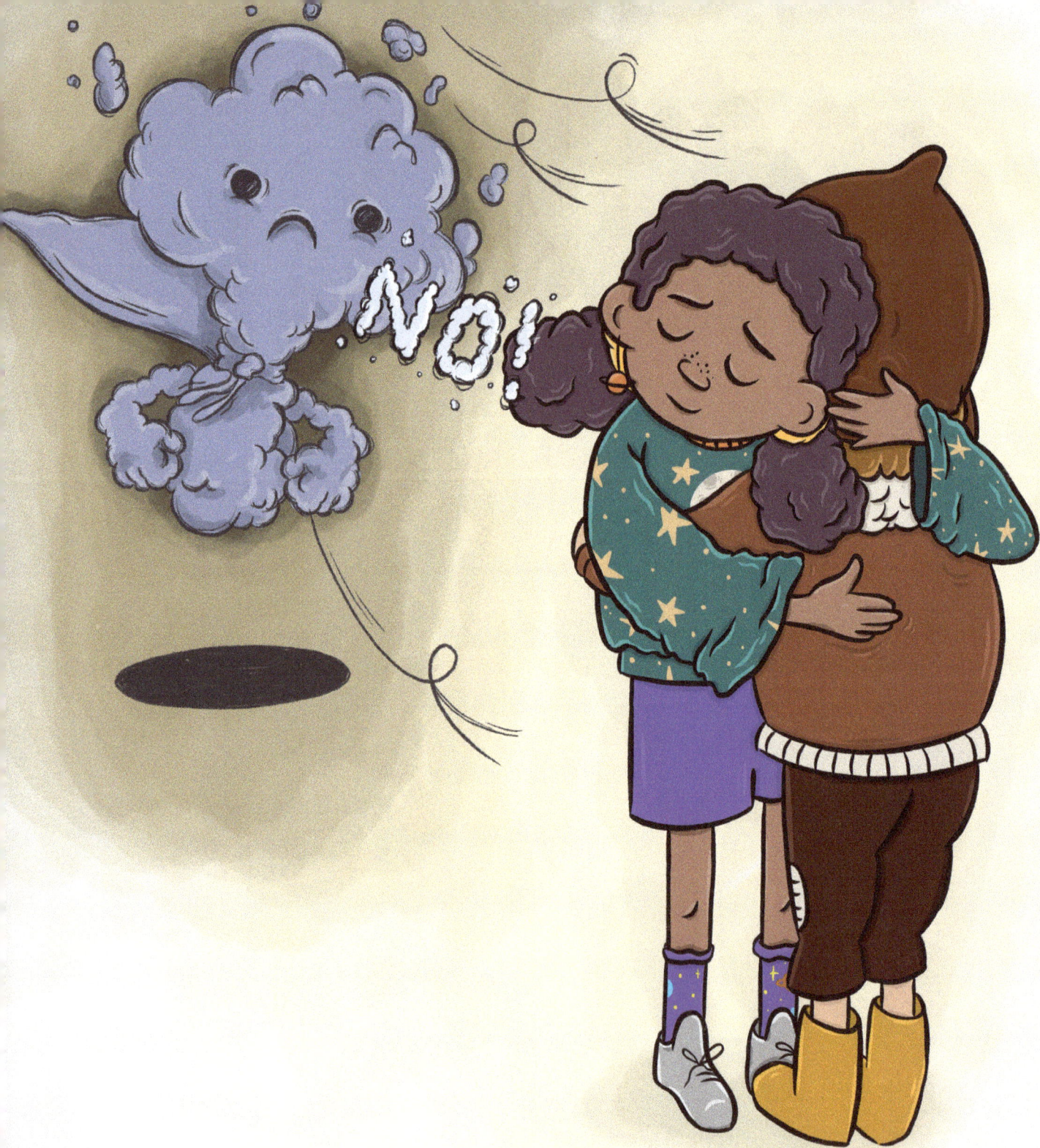

"Do you want to look through the telescope with me?" asks Amelia.

Her worry whisperer tells her **NO!**

– but Rosie decides to be brave.

She takes Amelia's hand and puts her eye to the eyepiece.

The universe unfolds around her like a sea of light. She sees galaxies bigger than anything she could ever imagine, and tiny grains of dust swirling around newborn stars. Space is so big, and she is so small.

Her worry whisperer is silent in awe.

"Daddy! Mummy!" Rosie cries.

"I'm not scared!"

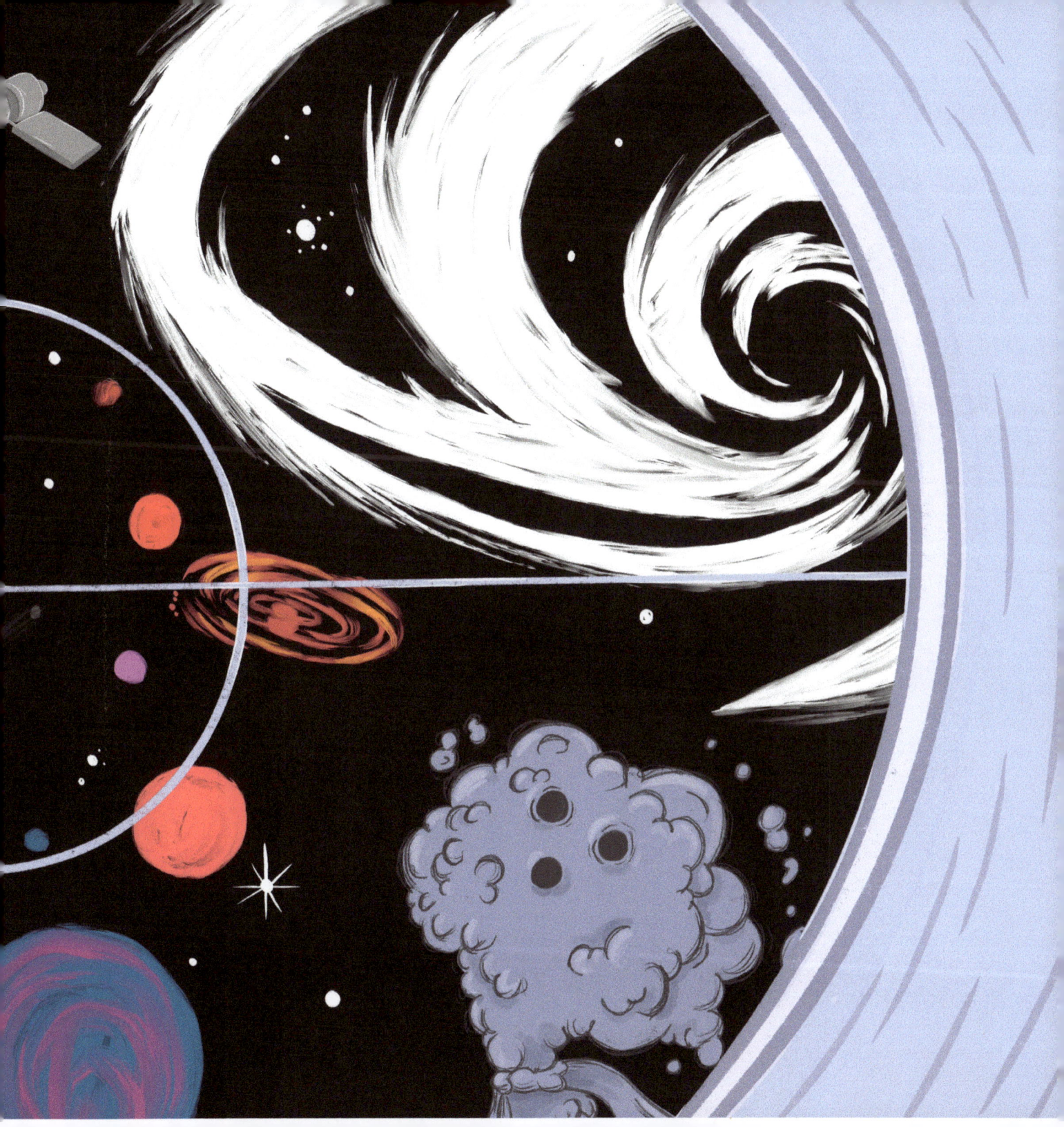

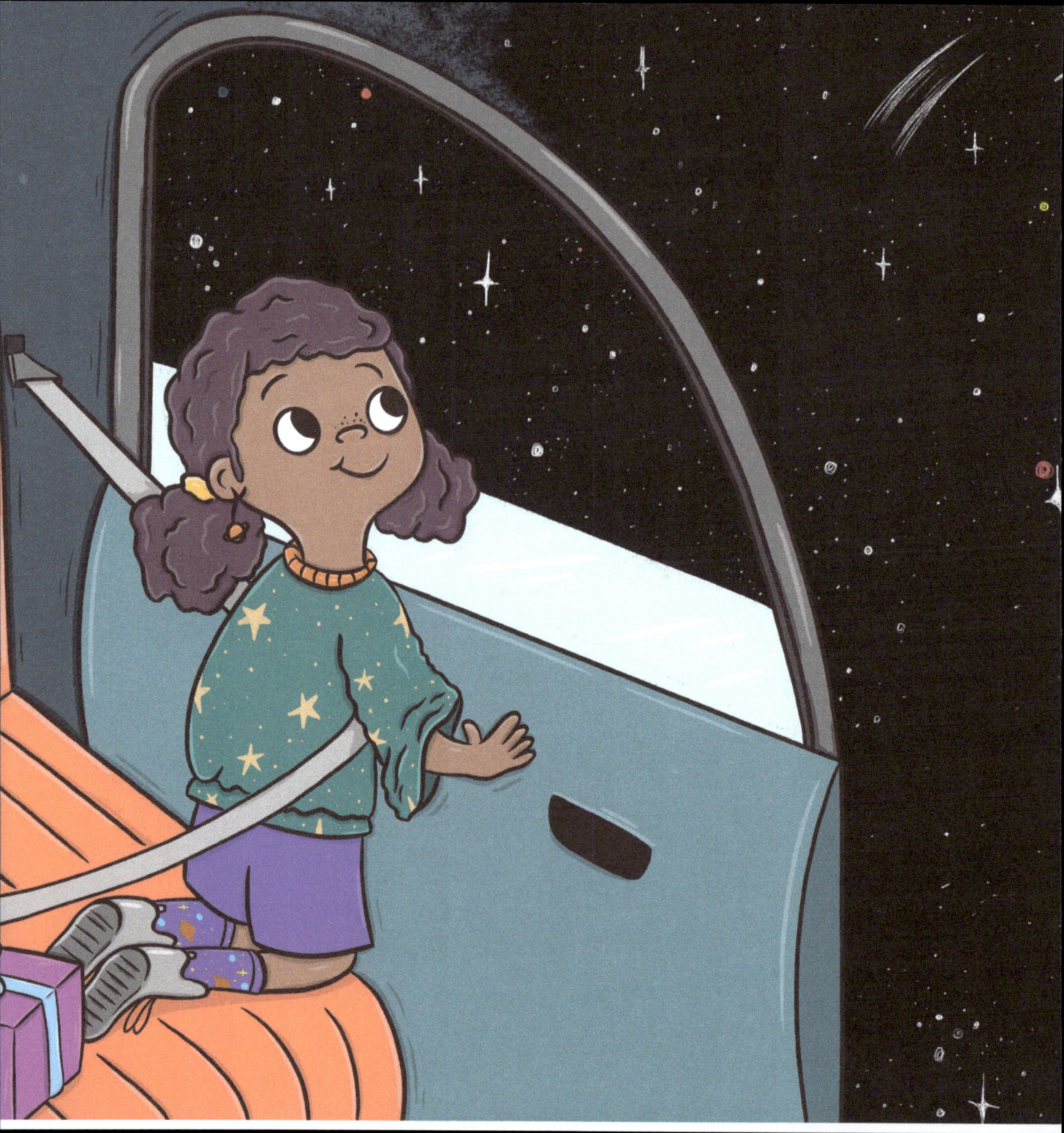

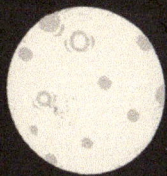

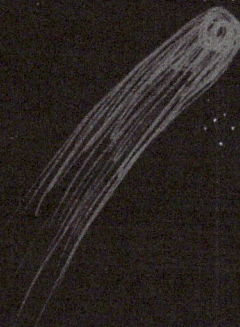

Rosie's worry whisperer is quiet on the drive home.

She knows that it will always be there to help keep her safe.

"But sometimes, it's okay not to listen to you," she whispers.

"Sometimes, I can be brave."

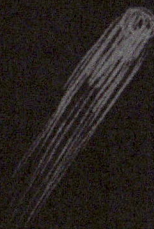

IP Kidz

an imprint of IP (Interactive Publications Pty Ltd)
Treetop Studio • 9 Kuhler Court
Carindale, Queensland, Australia 4152
ipoz.biz/ipstore

First published by IP in 2021

© 2021 Matthew Cunningham (text); Katharine Hall (illustrations)

ISBN 9781922332745 (HB); 9781922332752 (eBk)

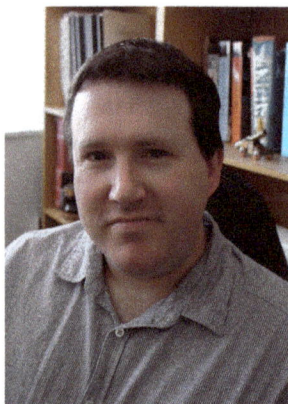

Matthew Cunningham is an author and historian based in the Greater Wellington region of Aotearoa New Zealand. He is the author of *Abigail and the Birth of the Sun,* which won Best Picture Book Award at the New Zealand Book Awards for Children and Young Adults 2020. He is currently working on two history books as well as his first full-length novel. Born in Australia, he now lives in Porirua with his wife and daughter Abigail, who, like her namesake, also likes to ask big questions.

Katharine Hall is an illustrator and graphic designer based in a small studio in Aotearoa. She tells stories that translate across language – specialising in ink work and digital design for individuals, start-ups, and businesses both big and small. Her third children's book was with Huia Publishing, her first being *Whetu toa and the Magician by Steph Matuku,* Winner of Storylines Notable Book Junior Fiction 2019 Award and New Zealand Book Award finalist. She is a graduate from Massey University with a Bachelor of Design (Hons) majoring in illustration.

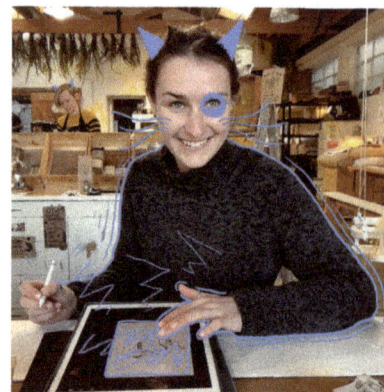

www.ingramcontent.com/pod-product-compliance
Lightning Source LLC
Chambersburg PA
CBHW041600260326
41914CB00011B/1336